RUNNING TOWARD TOMORROW

By

Maria M. Godwin

ISBN: 1-4033-2109-4 (e-book)
ISBN: 1-4033-2110-8 (Paperback)

This book is printed on acid free
paper.

1stBooks - rev. 07/19/02

CONTENTS

Acknowledgments
v

Introduction
ix

Chapter 1
1

Chapter 2
17

Chapter 3
31

Chapter 4
39

Chapter 5
94

Chapter 6
117

Epilogue
120

iii

ACKNOWLEDGMENTS

Before I started out on this project, I had it in my mind to write down all my inner thoughts and feelings about my treatments and how cancer affected my life. I never thought it was possible to actually sit down and take the time to write it as a book. Whether to have it published or to give as a gift of love to those who want to read it.

There are a number of special people who helped to make this book an inspirational passion for me. Without them I don't think I would have had the strength and courage to fight this illness, let alone be able to write about it for the benefit of others.

First, to my parents, family and friends, for all the inspiration, love, and prayers you send to help us keep our chins up high so that we can reach for the stars. Without you all, we couldn't have known the love and faith that helped keep us going.

To all the doctors and nurses who took special care of us. You are truly the Angels I needed to keep things in order when the difficulties of daily life became unbearable. Without you all, I wouldn't be alive today.

Finally, last but most definitely not forgotten. To my wonderful niece Hannah, for without her smiles I couldn't laugh. My cousin Marisa, for without her special prayers I couldn't believe, and most of all, my husband Joshua, for without his love and support I could not live. **I LOVE YOU! THANK YOU!** You have showed me how to live and most of all how to LOVE!

This book is dedicated to all cancer patients and their families. May God bless you and keep you all in the hearts and souls of your loved ones in your times of need. Whatever road you must travel remember this… you are never alone. There are always Angels there to guide you.

INTRODUCTION

I am writing this book to everyone who has been diagnosed with, or who knows someone battling cancer. There is no greater fear than the knowledge of knowing you must fight against a disease that can claim your life.

It is my hope that this book will give everyone who reads it a better understanding of what can happen to people when they are left to fight a deadly disease. Many things can change a person both, emotionally, physically, and spiritually.

This is my story, a story of my life, my experiences with the fight against neck and throat cancer. One of the more rare forms of cancer, which can hit middle age adults. To answer the biggest question everyone asks, no, I was not a smoker or a heavy drinker. Smoking and drinking has been linked to be a possible cause for this type of cancer. I share these experiences with you, as an insight, to help other people learn how I coped with one of life's deadly challenges.

I have come to learn for myself since being diagnosed with cancer, that there is no greater strength than the love and support of family, friends, and for me, my loving husband, Joshua.

My life was never easy. I don't believe that anyone can say his or her life is easy. Life doesn't come with any guarantees. You have to accept the cards you are dealt with and use them to your advantage. Life is what you make it out to be.

I grew up in a small town in Connecticut with my loving parents and younger sister. My parents and I haven't always seen many teenage topics eye-to-eye. Then again, when have you ever heard of a parent-teenager relationship that was completely flawless? Not! My sister and I were **very** different people. We grew up as your normal everyday siblings. We would tattle on each other, and beat each other up—literally. I was always on the losing end of the fight, but when your younger sister happens to be much bigger than you are, you can't help but lose a fight. As we got older we grew very far apart. We would do almost anything we could to avoid trying to communicate with each other.

Shortly after my eighteenth birthday, my grandfather passed away from lung cancer. His cancer had spread to his brain, and back then there wasn't much that could be done to save his life. I had never experienced death before. My grandfather's passing was the first in my family, and it affected me greatly.

Knowing he was dying of cancer, yet not knowing anything about the disease or what effects it had on people, was the hardest to deal with. I did as much research as I could about cancer and its affects on different people. I never found any literature regarding other people's experiences with this deadly disease. I felt useless not understanding the pain and emotional anguish my grandfather had gone through.

I learned from this point on what it was like to suffer through a loss. I had experienced the same thing that many people suffer through everyday. I was finally growing up and learning about life and death. What can destroy human life, as we know it; death is a difficult lesson to learn when you are a young teenager.

Life for me went down hill from there. I left home to find myself; my purpose for being alive in a world, that I felt, was cruel. I was in my senior year of high school, and working at the local fast food restaurant. I had no car, so that meant walking everywhere. I had my share of really bad experiences, and relationships. I learned the hard way about violence, abuse, and rape. I had tried to commit suicide several times, and couldn't seem to find that silver lining around that cloud.

Eventually, I found that silver lining. I graduated from high school, got a car, and a real job. My life was finally working out. I became, what I believed to be, a very strong, independent person who did her own thing. I had enough of bad relationships and wanted my life back. I depended on no one. I figured this would keep me from getting hurt. I had what I had, and it was all mine, if anyone pushed my buttons just right, they got the new me.

I was known to have a real bad attitude, and flared up temper. I wanted everyone to know I wasn't taking it anymore. No stepping on me, I could stand on my own two feet: even if they only had me standing four feet ten inches tall.

Little did I realize how much my life was about to change. I had an even bigger fight ahead of me. I had to fight for my will to **live.** A fight, that would change my whole perspective on how I viewed the world around me. I was about to experience a new outlook on life, and how important it is to live for today.

My motto through life has always been to believe in the magic of your dreams. If you have nothing to believe in you won't have any goals to strive for. For me, this seemed much easier said than done. I found it hard to have goals and dreams, only to watch them never happen.

As I have learned though, the only thing that is true in life, is no matter how much pain and suffering there may be in the world, we all touch the hearts, and have our hearts touched by many other people. Our existence touches the souls of every other person we come in contact with. Remember this: Life is like a mirror, so smile and see the whole world smiling right back at you.

The family I had a distant relationship with was about to show me that families are always there. They will always be my family, no matter what I have done to turn them away. The world I once knew as a cruel world would become a more beautiful world for me.

The ironic thing about my life, when I look back on it, is how I spent most of my teenage years trying to get out of my life, and now, I will be spending the rest of my life, fighting to stay alive.

My life experiences made me a strong believer of Angels. I believe there are always angels among us. We aren't always aware of their presence. It is believed that God sends us Angels during our most difficult times. I got the chance on several occasions, to open my heart and soul to see that my Angels came in many forms. I found for me, that God does love me, and doesn't wish bad things to happen to any of us. This doesn't mean bad things won't happen, but it does allow us the power of prayer. This is a power that can help us get closer to our beliefs, whatever they may be.

The story I am about to reveal to you is my life experience. I give to you this story in full. I give you all the wonderful, sad, difficult, and painful experiences. I hold nothing back.

I do this not for sympathy, not for pity. I do this in hope to touch your heart, and help you reach into your own soul. I hope this will make you see your world and understand how you can help comfort, or at least understand what can bring people together.

I ask that you open your hearts and minds, and realize that there is always someone out there that could use your love and support. No matter what the circumstances may be.

Cancer is a difficult disease to have. After all the treatment, pain, hurt, and sometimes, physical transformations, there come the very real memories, that will linger in ones mind for many years to come. Being able to be called, a SURVIVOR, is a very cherishable and monumental accomplishment.   So   these experiences, I give to you for strength and support in all your needs.

   This is my story...

CHAPTER 1

June 25, 1999, I was totally unaware of how much my life would change on this day.

I had gone to a local club, which was a local country dance bar and restaurant, to meet up with some friends. I had met the most incredible, unselfish, loving guy I had only been praying to find for so many years. His name was Joshua. He was intelligent, handsome, and fun. He was not like any other guy I had ever met.

I was working for a local phone company in Connecticut at the time, and he was in the military, stationed in Connecticut. We shared our first kiss on, June 26, 1999, our first actual date on June 27, 1999. I guess you could say this was love at first sight. Finally, I thought, this was the first time I had ever experienced the full meaning, of true love. This had been a very special weekend for me, and I was afraid that when the weekend ended, so would the relationship I was hoping to build on. I knew the possibility that this weekend would never happen again. Not with the one guy I thought was made for me, the match made in heaven.

It was Monday June 28, 1999, when I received a phone call. It was him, Josh, my dream guy from the weekend. He had been thinking of me as much as I was thinking about him. He asked me if we could meet somewhere, he wanted to see me. Josh and I spent the entire afternoon and well into the evening, on the beach close by the base.

We watched the most radiant sunset. The colors were so vibrant, and the breeze was blowing softly, and warm. There were boats sailing on the horizon that looked like soft silhouettes, sailing across the sky. The sounds of the waves splashing against the beach were carefree, and passionate. I felt as if I was caught in the most romantic dream, I was afraid to blink, with the thought of losing this romantic moment.

We knew then, that we were both very much in love. We couldn't dare think of a moment, that we wouldn't want to spend together. We talked about our family values, beliefs, and dreams. We realized we had more in common than we could ever have imagined. Dreaming about what it would be like to grow old together and have a family of our own. We dreamed about sitting in our rocking chairs on the front porch of our home, remembering all the good times we had. Our dreams were a part of our reality.

Speaking of reality, it was then that Josh told me about his transfer. He would be transferring to another military base—in Georgia. Together, we experienced a feeling of pain and hurt, believing that we may never see each other again. We then decided, it wasn't worth ruining what we had now, we would just make do with the time we had left. You know that old saying, <u>Cross that bridge when you come to it.</u>

Josh and I decided to move in together. It felt like the right thing to do. Josh had to learn to get along with the *other* man in my life, which was my 4-year-old, 130-pound Rottweiler whom I called Rox.

Rox was my long time companion and best friend. He was a very special part of my life. If I were crying, he would come up to me, and sit beside me and lick away my tears. He knew just what to do at the times I needed him most. It was no wonder that Josh and him got along so well. Rox must have felt that Josh and him were there for the same reasons, which were to protect me, and be there to love me.

On July 22, 1999, I had come home late after working a double shift. I was not surprised to find Josh and Rox asleep on the living room sofa. However, I was surprised to see a small, crushed-velvet box sitting on Josh's chest. I reached over to grab it, when Josh took my hand, sat up, and in an almost slow, yet smooth motion, he got down on one knee, and asked me if I would be his wife. The emotions of that moment, just poured out all at once. The tears just flowed down my face like a smooth warm rain. I could hardly believe that someone loved me that much to ask me to be there wife. Of course, I said, YES!

Within the next couple of days, we notified our parents about the engagement. He did do the proper thing, Josh asked my father for his blessing, to which my parents said they were hoping this would happen. They knew Josh and I were meant to be together. They were very happy for the both of us.

Josh grew up in a small town in Texas with his parents and younger brother. When we met I was twenty-nine, and Josh was nineteen. Mind you, the age factor played no part on our relationship. We loved each other just the same.

The funny thing was, we had only three weeks to plan our wedding. My family stepped in and offered to help. Everything would be taken care of. Josh and I only had to get our blood work done and arrange some small, minor details.

It was while having my blood work done for the wedding, that I realized I had a lump on the left side of my neck. I mentioned it to my doctor, and he prescribed antibiotics. This wasn't at all alarming to me, since I was used to getting what are known as cysts, from time to time. I had noticed, after finishing the medicine the lump was still there. I figured, since I felt no pain, there was no need for worry at that time. Besides, I had a wedding to plan, and another tragedy I was, unknowingly, going to have to face.

It was on August 18, 1999, two days before our wedding. I had to bring my dog, Rox, over to the veterinarian. It seemed Rox was very ill. I was terrified and unsure what to do. The test results showed that my dog, Rox, had a disease that was known as a dormant blood disease. It was inherited, and no one knew he had it. Unfortunately, something caused the disease to become active. The disease was terminal.

My best friend was dying and there wasn't anything; anyone could do for him. I refused to believe this. When he was only six months old he was infected with the parvovirus, and almost died. My dog miraculously survived. He was my little miracle, and I wanted to believe he would beat this disease also. When I got home later that day I told everyone who knew Rox and loved him, what was happening. There were a lot of tears shed, worrying about what was going to happen to him.

The hardest challenge in my life at this point was, knowing that I was going to lose my best friend. Josh was very supportive for me, knowing that Rox was going to die. We could only be with him, and love him until that time came for him to leave us.

The other hardest challenge was moving out of Connecticut, where I spent all my life growing up and making friends. Josh was very supportive of this transition also. The best part was, knowing I was going to be the wife of a great man. We knew we were made to be together.

On August 21, 1999, Joshua and I were married. It was a beautiful day, although it was pouring cats and dogs outside, and our reception ended up in a garage. With family and friends, it turned out to be a very special day. Even Josh's mom, dad, and brother came to Connecticut, from Texas, to be with us on our special day. It was funny to imagine how a "good-old-country-boy" from Texas could end up falling in love with a "smart-mouthed-Italian girl" from Connecticut. Reminds me of, <u>The West Side Story.</u> Anyway, I thank God every day for bringing my husband into my life.

A week after our wedding, Josh and I had to say goodbye to our family and friends in Connecticut, and start our journey towards our new life together. It was hard to say goodbye; there were many tears and sad faces. One of the most difficult good-byes for me was to my best friend, Lisa, and my little cousin Marisa. The most heart-wrenching good-byes were to my mom and dad, and my niece, Hannah. Oh, how I love my Hannah-bell.

Josh and I were on our journey towards our new life. I had my dog, Rox, in the backseat of my car, and we followed behind Josh in his truck. We were heading to Josh's hometown in Texas. There we would spend some time with his family and friends. There was a hurricane in Georgia, and the military base had been evacuated.

This not only gave Josh a chance to introduce me to his family and friends, but also allowed us some extra time for him to show me where he grew up.

Texas was beautiful. Josh's family gave us a warm welcome, and threw us an old-fashion Texas reception to celebrate our wedding. I must admit Texas was very different for me than Connecticut. No trees out there just flat land and dirt roads that went on for miles. The most exciting thing for me was the storms. Having lived in Connecticut most of my life, there is nothing that compares to a Texas thunder storm. The first storm I got to watch was incredible. The night was pitched black, and the air was comfortably warm. The breeze felt like a light mist off an ocean wave. The lightning was so vivid you could make out all the jagged lines, and so bright that in the dark of night you could see every road, every house, and make out every little detail. The best part was there wasn't any rain. It was so romantic and peaceful to sit out on the porch, and watch the heat storm in all its fury.

Within a couple of weeks, my dog, Rox, was actually running around and looking very happy. It was amazing, how he just perked up full of life all of a sudden. It was refreshing for me to see him running after Josh and me in the yard. He must have been getting better, or so I was hoping.

One morning, shortly thereafter, Josh and I got up to go meet some of his friends for the day. I looked at Rox, and he didn't seem right. I had an awful feeling wrenching into my stomach. I just knew something was really wrong. Josh convinced me that he would be okay after he rested up awhile, so we left. When we got home in the early evening Josh's parents explained to me that Rox hadn't eaten anything all day, and wouldn't move. I rushed to his side, and saw he wasn't doing well. Josh got him some water and he drank, barely being able to hold up his head.

That evening looked to storm again, I told Josh I was going to spend some time with Rox. I went outside and rested his head in my lap. I spoke to him for almost two hours. His eyes looked very tired. I sat there crying telling him it was okay to let go. Soon after, I got him to come into the garage. I laid out his favorite blanket for him and told him that I loved him very much. I leaned down to his face, and he gave me a kiss.

Later that night I had a vision that Rox had wings. He was healthy, happy, and barking at me as if I was holding up a T-bone steak. The next morning I woke up with the eerie feeling of loss and emptiness. I went to the garage and before I could open the door, an uneasy feeling came over me. As I stepped into the garage, the smell of death was in the air; it was then that I realized Rox had passed away. When I reached out my hand to touch his head, he was very cold, I knew he had been dead for awhile. Maybe he died after kissing me goodnight, or was that his final kiss goodbye? I guess I will never know.

My father-in-law dug the grave out back for Rox. Josh brought me up to the canyon to find some rocks we could place around his grave. We also went and bought some silk flowers to place by the tombstone that Josh made him. Oh how Rox loved to smell flowers. He was a very different type of dog.

Josh took the time to carve his name into a piece of flat marble, which made up his tombstone. Beneath his name were the words: "pooh-bear", which was the nickname I gave him long ago. Losing Rox almost seemed unfair. My mother advised me of something I never realized; she told me that when Rox came into my life, I was in need of a friend, someone I could count on to be with me.

When my husband Josh and I got married, Rox knew that his job here on Earth, with me, was done. Rox knew that Josh was going to be the one who would be there for me now, and it was time for him to go back home, with the Angels. Rox was my guardian angel throughout his life. Without my special friend I would not have made it through some of my toughest moments. Rest in Peace my friend. I will love and miss you always.

Maria M. Godwin

On September 29, 1999, we packed up our belongings and were heading out to the military base in Georgia. This is where we would start our new, wonderful life together. I took a few moments to say goodbye to Rox's grave, knowing his spirit will always be with me.

On our journey to Georgia, I had a very bad sore throat. I almost felt like it was swelling a little, but as before, I passed it off as a nervous reaction, due to our leaving the stability we had in Texas for the unknown we would face in Georgia.

CHAPTER 2

On October 1, 1999, Josh and I arrived in Georgia. Within a few hours we were checked into the base, and had found an apartment close by that we could call home. We knew it was going to be difficult at first trying to adjust to new people and a different environment. Not having any friends, and no job, I knew it wasn't going to be easy on me. The different changes were causing Josh and I to feel very stressed about life. We knew we had to pull together through these difficult times, and help each other cope with our new lifestyle together, as a couple.

The first decision we made, was compromise on a church we could attend. With us both having different religious backgrounds, yet believing in the same things, we decided on an Episcopal church in town. This little church had such a warm and down home southern feeling, that we knew right away, this was our church.

In no time at all, we were making friends and meeting people, and soon, I had finally found a job. Our lives were once again starting to come together the way we wanted it to be, in perfect harmony. We were very thankful for all the positive things that were entering into our lives; we were finally starting to feel like a family.

The first neighbors we met became our very best friends. They lived upstairs from us and were wonderful neighbors. Paul is in the military with Josh, and Lizzy is a homemaker with their young son, Adam. I was finally at peace with myself about our life together, and we are very much in love. Nothing could go wrong. We are the fairy tale couple who will live happily-ever-after.

On October 3, 1999, I wasn't feeling very well. Josh took me to the medical clinic. I had a slight sore throat and Josh was beginning to worry about the lump in my neck that still hadn't gone away. The doctor had decided it would be best to send me to an Ear, Nose, and Throat specialist, for further evaluation. My appointment for the specialist was made for October 29. I figured that was fine since the pain was tolerable.

On October 27,1999, just two days before my appointment with the specialist for my throat, I woke up very sick. My head was throbbing, my ears were ringing, and my throat was swollen. As the day went on I was having more trouble swallowing. By that evening Josh was so concerned he brought me to the local hospital emergency room. There the doctors prescribed a pain medication called Darvacet, and 800 milligrams of Motrin. This was to help stop the swelling and the pain in my throat.

The only trouble I was having with all this medication was that I was only weighing in at about eighty-five pounds; soak-and-wet. The emergency room doctors had made their diagnosis of, swollen glands and an infection that had looked to resemble tonsillitis. Later that evening, I was stable enough to be sent home.

The following morning, not more than eight hours later, I was rushed back to the emergency room. It seemed the medication wasn't working fast enough, and the swelling in my throat had gotten worse. I was running a fever of 102, and I started having severe pain in my left eye. I apparently was swallowing thick mucus from the infection in my throat, which seemed to be causing me to vomit violently.

I was taken in immediately. The nurses put an intravenous tube (IV) into my arm in case my breathing became shallow. Within twenty minutes, the doctors decided to give me a medicine to relax my muscles through my IV tube to relieve the swelling in my throat more quickly, as well as a medication to control the vomiting. Four hours later the nurse said my condition was stable, and I could go home... again.

The next morning I had my appointment with the Ear, Nose, and Throat Specialist. I was on so much medication to help control the pain and swelling at this time, that Josh had to walk with me. I couldn't find the strength or energy to stand, let alone get up and walk.

The doctor saw that my throat was very swollen. She had to use a special device that goes through the nostril of your nose, and is guided through the nose, down into the back of the throat. This device was specially made so the doctors could see inside your throat without you having the feeling of gagging or choking. You think the procedure sounds gross, HA! Not only that, but it was very uncomfortable!

The procedure showed the doctor that my tongue had aspirated. This meant that part of my tongue had blistered and split open, causing a very bad infection. I was taken off the Motrin, which was relaxing the muscles in my throat, and I was put on an antibiotic to fight the infection. I was then instructed to return to the ENT Specialist's office for further evaluation, after the medication was completed.

Two weeks later, when I returned, there was no infection. I was able to open my mouth and talk normally again without pain. Except for the swelling in my neck, I was feeling pretty good. The doctor made the decision to keep me on the antibiotic a few days longer, so we could keep the infection from returning until we could find what was causing the aspiration. I was still taking Darvacet, as needed to regulate the pain.

The next step is to have a procedure done that was known as a CAT Scan with contrast of the neck and throat. In case you are unaware of this procedure, I'll explain. The nurses put an IV tube into your arm and slowly add a dye, otherwise known as "contrast." The dye is rather unique. You see, the nurse warns you ahead of time that you will feel your body start to get very warm, then you will feel as if you are wetting your pants.

The nurse told me about a patient they had, who really thought they were wetting their pants and took off running down the hallway for the bathroom. That made me laugh, hysterically. The thought that I was "wetting" my pants, after a few minutes they start to take x-rays. The contrast actually helps them see any abnormalities a little clearer. When the entire process is done, usually about twenty minutes, you can sit up… slowly. In a minute or two, you are as good as new. I'll tell you, that this was definitely an interesting experience.

Within a few days, I was back in the specialist's office to get the results of the scan. She was very thorough in explaining to me what she was seeing. I was grateful for the fact that she was using terminology I was able to understand. The scan showed that there was a mass in my neck on the left side, about the size of a half-dollar. She also noted another mass seen on my tongue, which was the size of a nickel. The mass in my neck was attached to a lymph node, and some nerves, which was causing my pain.

The next step was to have a needle biopsy done. A biopsy is done to collect any fluid, preferably, cells. This way they can test them for abnormalities. Doing this procedure would help to determine the best means of treatment. The biopsy would be performed on the cyst in my neck, which the doctor believes is the "secondary" mass. This mass was much easier to reach to perform this type of procedure. Within a few minutes she was on the phone calling in the pathologist who was at the medical center close by. Mind you I was in no hurry for him to get here. Unfortunately Josh had to work that day, and was unable to be there for my appointment.

The pathologist came in and explained the procedure to me. Somehow, I was so nervous, (I **HATE** needles), that I must have taken what he was saying to me and let it go in one ear and out the other. All I heard was… needle… few minutes. So my thought was, ok, no problem, I can handle this. YEAH RIGHT was I ever **DEAD WRONG!**

The first part of the procedure is to sterilize my neck with iodine and alcohol. My nervousness had completely taken over my body now. The next step is to use a ballpoint pen to mark where the needle would enter into the cyst. My exact thought at this moment was more like… **GET ME OUT OF HERE!!!** He then proceeded to reach for the needle, to which, I kid you not, was made for a HORSE! He stuck the needle into the cyst and pulled out what he called cells. For me… the procedure felt more like he was sucking out my brain. **OUCH! PAIN, PAIN, PAIN!** Feel free to cringe… I did.

Finally, the cells were on their way to their next destination, a slide that he put under a microscope. Then he added some purple dye to them to make them glow. Unaware to me, but very believable, after he looked at the slide through his microscope, he had very bad news; the first needle didn't collect enough cells for him to make the procedure work! The pathologist had to stick me again, with the **HORSE** needle! Let me try to explain the PAIN I was feeling at this point, **EXCRUCIATING!!!** I do believe this about sums it all up… don't you?

Again, after a few days, I was back in the specialist's office where she explained the results of the needle biopsy to both Josh and I. Apparently the biopsy showed many "infected" cells. Proper diagnosis was still not possible. The biopsy results were unable to obtain the abnormal cells origin, there were still not enough cells collected.

Let me just say that my reaction went somewhat like this: Not enough cells? You've got to be kidding! You STUCK me twice, and made me feel like you were sucking out my BRAINS! All this and all you have to say is… **NOT ENOUGH CELLS!!! Tough! Too bad! You're not getting anymore! No way! Out of the question! Don't even think about it!**

After that small, yet sudden act of hysteria, the doctor advised me of our next step towards finding out what these abnormal cells were, and how we could treat them. This procedure was known as a surgical biopsy. The surgical biopsy involved going after cells from the primary mass that was located at the base of my tongue. This would involve taking and cutting out a small piece of the mass, and putting it under a microscope to find the origin.

Here we go again! And to think I was just saying to myself, that I haven't had any excitement in my life in about a day or be two. This will be so much fun! Yeah right! I more or less wanted to run and hide instead of being put under a knife— thank you very much! Mind you, at this stage in the game, a little sarcasm should be expected. Helps with the issue of SANITY!

Needless to say, I went home that night and didn't sleep very well. I need some kind of *PEACE*. I found the power of PRAYER really works for me.

A few nights before the biopsy, I had a dream. My grandfather came to me; he told me that I had cancer. I spent time in my dream crying to him. He told me to be strong.

CHAPTER 3

On December 16, 1999, Josh took me to the local hospital again to prepare for the procedure. I went into the room, and they had me put on a cap and gown and these awful, non-traditional, booties. The nurse came in and hooked me up to an IV unit for fluids.

The pastor of our church, Father Mac, as he liked to be called, came to see Josh and me before the procedure. We all said a little prayer together. The prayer really made me feel better. Soon after they put a sleeping medication into my IV tube, within a few minutes, it was lights out.

When I finally awoke in the recovery room I became instantly aware that, HEY, I wasn't in any pain. NO pain, YES this was great!

Oh, what a blessing! Then I noticed Josh was standing besides me, with tears in his eyes. Apparently Father Mac and Josh were already told the news.

When I became more alert the doctor came in to discuss the prognosis with me. She advised me... I had malignant cancer. She said this type of cancer is usually seen in men over the age of sixty-five, who have smoked or chewed tobacco all their lives. It was rare to find this cancer in someone my age, (mind you, I was only 29 at this time and didn't smoke, or chew tobacco for that matter).

Okay... my reaction? Well lets just say I wasn't asking why I had it, or even saying why me? I guess that "Tough Cookie, Very Independent, I can handle anything," attitude just took over again. I was actually very calm and very aware what I had. (I remembered, a little birdie told me). My only question was what do we do now? The doctors made it very clear to me up front: you fight and do treatment; you can win, you give up and refuse treatment; you will *definitely* die.

I thought I was aware of what was in store for me. I thought I was aware of how to fight and win the battle, over this deadly disease. My strength was definitely going to be put to the test.

I think one of the toughest things Josh and I had to do, was tell our families. Most people look at cancer as the disease that causes people to die. The last thing I wanted my family to feel was hurt because of me. Josh was very supportive in helping me tell my family, and then he told his. I had a strong belief that with the power of prayer, and my loving husband, I would beat this disease. One way or another I was going to give it my ALL! I refuse to be another victim of cancer.

The Sunday following the diagnosis Josh and I decided to go to our church service. We needed to find some kind of peace. During each service Father Mac makes the weekly announcements. He stood up, and to our surprise, he advised everyone to keep Josh and I in his or her prayers. He went on to inform everyone that I was diagnosed with malignant cancer.

The part that touched my heart the most was when Father Mac stated that with both Josh and I having family out of state, they all wanted us to know that everyone in our church is our family too. They would be there for support and prayers to both of us during this difficult journey that lied ahead. I know this brought tears and much needed comfort to both Josh and me.

It was at this time, I met my wonderful friend, Rosina. Rosina is a remarkable person. She balances her life like everyone else: job, husband, and two wonderful kids. She is also a cancer survivor of several years. Although Rosina's cancer experience would be quite different from mine; she is a gem of a friend. With a promise to have a cup of coffee waiting, she is always there to lend a helping hand. Whether I need to talk, or just need a shoulder to cry on, Rosina was always there.

The next morning Josh and I awoke to start our trip to Connecticut. Against the doctor's advice, Josh was taking me home to see my family and friends for Christmas. We didn't know when I would be able to come back home to see my family, so before treatment started, we wanted to get in a quiet vacation.

I knew that this holiday wasn't going to be as cheerful as we wanted, but we would all be together. I saw the pain in my mom and dad's eyes. All I could do to keep from crying was to just try and have a nice holiday. The best and most painful part for me was looking at my twenty-three months old niece, Hannah, and seeing her beautiful smile. I love the way she runs to me and gives me a hug. The way she says Wuv E. Spending this time with my family made me realize the possibility that I may never see them again if I don't do what needs to done to treat this illness. Well this made me more determined to win the fight.

Overall, going back home for Christmas and seeing my family and friends made me look at many things differently. Everything looked a little fresher. The grass was a shade of green I had never seen before. The sky was a shade of blue I had never noticed. The clouds seemed fluffy, and even the flowers smelled sweeter. It is truly amazing how many things we take for granted when we are in a hurry to get through each day. Funny how being sick can change your perspective on how you view the little things. It is sad to see that an illness has to open people's hearts and minds a little more.

I know that Christmas is a time for love, family, and friends. I was determined to make the best of this holiday season. I have to admit God does work in mysterious ways. My mom and I are very close. We always have been, and I know deep in my heart we will stay this way. My dad and I never could quite see eye-to-eye on anything but we managed to set aside our differences. I guess you could say I have my father's stubborn pride. The relationship I share with my father now, is one I will cherish forever. As for my sister and me, well like I said, we are very different on how we view things, but she's not so bad after all. Since being diagnosed with cancer, we have been a loving and caring family, without the bitterness.

CHAPTER 4

January of 2000, the new Millennium has arrived. It is funny how most people are home, worrying about the Y2K bug causing major malfunction in the world. Meanwhile, Josh and I were back home in Georgia, celebrating our first New Year's together. With just the two of us, and a romantic candlelight dinner. Besides, the worries on our mind are more in the thought of what is going to happen to me, and how we were going to deal with it. This will be a real life challenge and it scared us to death. We vowed to each other to stay strong for one another as best as we could.

On January 4, 2000, I was sent to another doctor, an oncologist who specialized in neck and throat cancer. The oncologist reviewed my case and explained everything to Josh and me.

The first plan of attack is for me to start radiation treatment first. The size of the tumor on my tongue is so large, that if he were to remove the tumor surgically; he would have to remove such a large portion of my tongue. Thus making it necessary to remove the esophagus and voice box as well, to keep me from choking.

The oncologist felt that for my age removing all of this would only be as a last resort, if all else failed. He also stated that if the radiation kills this tumor I would have a better chance to live my life as normal as possible. This was news that terrified me more than any other. The thought of losing my ability to ever speak again is a thought I couldn't bear think about. This is when I realized how the words I use to express my emotions need to be very delicate. The way we speak makes a great impact on our lives. I wasn't ready to lose my ability to speak. **EVER!**

The tumor in my neck is another problem. This tumor will require surgery to remove it. The doctor said that no matter what the radiation does this tumor would need to be removed. Apparently, this tumor decided to attach itself to the lymph node on that side of my throat. The problem we face here is that the doctor won't know without surgery whether this tumor has invaded an artery, veins, or nerve. Finally, we don't know how far into the lymph node this tumor has spread.

The lymph node has several layers to it. The way the doctors tell if the cancer has spread into other parts of the body is to see how far into the lymph node it has traveled. The surgical procedure is known as lymphatic dissection. Basically, this is the removal of all the lymph node until they clean out all the cancer. If they don't get it all this runs the risk of the cancer possibly spreading to major organs throughout my body.

I have to say that this started looking more serious than I expected. I guess I was figuring on a little operation and healing time and I would be getting back to my life with my husband. I never realized, or maybe I didn't want to realize, just how bad this could be. Again, I wanted to run and hide, or maybe cry this all away. I knew now, there was no place for me to hide. I have to face this head on… like it or not.

The next thing the oncologist wanted to talk to us about was just as bad as having cancer. This wasn't a topic up for discussion either. He advised us of the importance of having a feeding tube put in place (temporarily) to help aid in my nutritional intake. He said what would happen is the radiation to my facial area and throat will cause severe burns and blistering. This problem will keep me from being able to eat, so with the feeding tube in place I can still get my nutrition.

By the time we were ready to leave the oncologist's office, I was so numb I don't know how I got to the parking lot. I'm sure Josh took hold of me, otherwise I would have surely fallen.

I couldn't help but think my life was falling apart again. Only this time I wasn't hurting myself, I was hurting my husband as well. I wanted so much not to hurt him this way. I felt so bad I thought for sure that he wouldn't want to be with me anymore.

The following week I had an appointment with the general surgeon who would be putting in the feeding tube. The surgeon explained how they would make an incision just above the navel, cutting up about two or three inches. Then the surgeon would be cutting a small hole to the left of the incision to place the tube in. The tube would then be guided through the two-inch incision to my stomach; there he will make a small incision and insert the tube. The tube would be kept in place by a rubber balloon, filled with water inside my stomach to keep it in place.

The thought of having a tube sticking out of my stomach about a foot long, wasn't exactly what I had in mind. The thought of the scars this was going to leave behind really made me feel ugly inside. I couldn't help but think if I was ever going to wear a two-piece bathing suit again without all these ugly scars. Isn't it kind of funny how you worry about the little things, like appearance?

I think it is here that I should point out that the military is aware of my health condition. Josh made it a point to let them know what was happening. They were very concerned. They granted Josh his request to stay by my side for as long as he needed. This made me feel much better knowing my husband is going to be able to be with me through this difficult time.

January 13, 2000, (no not Friday, thank goodness) Josh took me to a hospital in Florida, where they will be doing my surgery.

He went to admissions to check me in while I waited in the waiting room. I will be spending the next few days in the hospital following my surgery. Yet again, I got to put on a little cap and gown and those horrible looking booties.

Shortly before I was brought in for Surgery, Rosina and a Deacon from our church came to pray with Josh and I. I want to say that I felt better, but I can't lie. I was very glad to say a prayer, however, I can't oversee the fact that I am so scared, and afraid that I will never wake up.

When surgery was over I was taken to my room on a wing known as Four Central. I could have never imagined the excruciating pain you get when your abdominal muscles have been cut. I was unable to sit up, walk, cough, or laugh. I couldn't even roll over or lift my head off the pillow. The pain was so unbearable the doctor put me on a Morphine drip. I can say on several occasions I didn't remember much at all. I only know that I was able to hit the button for the Morphine every twelve minutes. I do believe I hit it every chance I got.

At this time I was being introduced to another wonderful person, thanks to Rosina. Her name is Maryanne. Maryanne is a spiritual person. More so than I could ever see myself being. She came to sit with me, and read Psalms to me, in an effort to subside my fears and make me feel better. I came to find a particular Psalm that I enjoyed very much. I made myself a promise that whenever I got scared or started to lose my faith, I would recite this Psalm. It brought me to the point of peace that I needed. Helping me to find the courage and the strength to get me through whatever might be troubling me at the time. Fear was becoming my newfound friend and I looked for this Psalm to bring my faith back to God.

My favorite Psalm is known as:

A Psalm of David

The Lord is my shepherd, I shall not
want
He maketh me to lie down in green
pastures.
He leadeth me beside the still
waters.
He restoreth my soul.
He leadeth me in the path of
Righteousness for his Names sake.
Yea, though I walk through the
valley of the shadow of Death,
I will fear no evil, for thou art
with me,
Thy rod and thy staff they comfort
me.
Thou preparest a table before me in
the presence of mine enemies.
Thou anointed my head with oil.
My cup runneth over.
Surely, goodness and mercy shall
follow me all the days of my life,
and I will dwell in the house of the
Lord forever.

-Psalm 23

This is the Psalm that brings me
the peace, and the serenity I need to
find my strength in the deepest, and
the darkest moments. I am thankful
everyday to be so blessed with the

knowledge and belief in the Power of Prayer, to use this power as my guide to help me in times of need. It always brought me to the point of peace that I needed. Helping me to find the courage and the strength and get me through whatever might be troubling me.

Rosina and Maryanne came to see me in the hospital several times. Maryanne wanted to pray with me. I was in so much pain at times that I found it very difficult to focus on anything. This is when she felt I needed her the most.

Maryanne definitely has a healing warmth to her touch. She helped me to focus so I could concentrate on feeling better, instead of feeling hurt, and upset over the surgery and how helpless I felt to myself and my husband.

The nurses on my floor were also very exceptional people. I met one nurse who was terrific. She was so understanding and caring I will never forget the kindness she showed me. Her nickname for me… kitten. She said I reminded her of a small and fragile kitten. She always had a warm glow to her, kind of like an Angel in disguise.

I also met another nurse who loved to make everyone smile. He was a male nurse who would come in and sit with Josh and me. The two of them would tell jokes back and forth, and Josh would tease me saying I probably liked having a male nurse. I kept screaming at them both, telling them to stop making me laugh since it hurt so much to laugh. You know how men can be when they get going with a few good jokes.

Finally, I come to a nurse who would come and visit me all the time even if I wasn't her patient. She always made it a point to see me at least once everyday to see if I needed anything. Most of all, I had my wonderful husband. He stayed overnight, every night, sleeping in a lounge chair in my room, right up next to my bed. Josh never left my side. He always took special care of me. If he had to go somewhere he would always be sure to let the nurses know I would be alone for awhile.

Several days after my surgery I was taken off the Morphine. The pain was still very severe, but I would be going home soon, and this meant it was time to find another form of pain control.

After discontinuing the Morphine I started running high fevers and getting very sick. I even started with fever blisters in my mouth. The doctors were unsure of what was causing this.

I finally got to go home, I was still running a fever and very sick. The doctors said this might be a withdrawal reaction caused by the Morphine, in this case I would just have to wait it out. I was sent home with another pain medication known as Percocet. I wasn't home for more than three hours when I started vomiting violently. I couldn't keep anything down, including water. I was like this for five days before the vomiting finally eased up. I was very dehydrated and weak, but I was able to start getting some real food down.

Ten days after my surgery, I was still in pain. I couldn't walk without assistance, and was sleeping on our couch in the living room propped up on pillows. Josh spent the last several days crunched up on the loveseat next to me, he said in case

I needed him during the night; he wanted to be close by.

While I was still unable to move well, I went to meet with my radiation therapist. He would be responsible for calculating how much radiation I will need as well as for how long. The radiation therapist took one look at me and said that I must get my strength back before radiation treatments started. He said that the radiation itself would cause me to become very ill, and weak. It was important that I get plenty of rest and eat as much as possible to build up my strength. (Little did I realize how right he would be)?

The next day I went to the treatment center to be fitted for my very own mask. They said that a mesh mask would be made to help them line up the radiation beams that they would be using to zap the cancer. I will have markings on my chest across my collarbone, and markings on the mask. The mask fit very snug over my head and face.

In a few days I started my radiation treatments. I would lie down on my back on a hard, cold, fiberglass table. The nurses would place the mask over my face, the mask is mesh, so I can see and breathe. The mask is then BOLTED down with screws to the table to lock my head in place. The mask covered my whole head and came down about two inches from my chin.

I must say, please don't try this stunt at home. I also don't recommend this for anyone who is claustrophobic either. The radiation beams start on the right side of my face and neck for about forty-five seconds, then the beams are moved to the left side of my face and neck for the same length of time. After a few seconds the machine is placed above me so the beams will be hitting me directly on my face. I get hit from all possible angles in order to make sure we kill the tumors.

My scheduled treatments would begin on January 26, 2000, and run Monday through Friday for ten weeks. The actual radiation treatment itself doesn't hurt. The mask is very uncomfortable but the treatment is like having an x-ray done.

February 4, 2000. I celebrated my 30th birthday. Josh bought me four beautiful balloons, roses, and a giant teddy bear for me to hold when he couldn't be with me. (Which mind you, wasn't very often.) The card, I treasure the most. His words were so romantic and full of passion. Telling me that he will always love me and be here for me.

Unfortunately, I celebrate my birthday while going through

radiation treatment. All the nurses sang happy birthday and tried to make this day as nice as possible. You know what? It was a beautiful day. It was a special day. I am a year older.

All the doctors and nurses at the treatment center are always willing to sit and talk with Josh and me. They are concerned with our emotions and how we are feeling.

It did take me almost an hour to eat the cupcake I got for my birthday, but I was devoted to getting that cupcake down no matter how much it hurt my mouth and throat to eat it. Besides, you only turn 30 once.

It didn't take long before I started feeling the effects of the radiation. I would leave a session, and about two hours later would be very feverish and ill. I started feeling like I was in a large microwave oven.

The tumor on my tongue was starting to react to the radiation. The tumor got so angry, it started swelling which then aggravated the tumor in my neck. Together the tumors decided to retaliate. **Against ME!** I started with severe pain in my left ear, head, and left eye. The radiation is even affecting my night vision terribly too. I became super sensitive to sunlight, and bright lights. I felt like I was turning into a creature of the night.

Soon after this, the radiation started causing some bad mouth sores. I was experiencing such severe pain in my mouth and throat that I became unable to drink water. The water felt like razor blades going down my throat. As fast as I sipped the water was as fast as the tears were running down my face. Again, my positive attitude is being tested. Little did I realize by this point in time that this was still only the beginning of the fight I was going to have to go through.

The power of prayer; what a powerful phrase this is. I prayed a lot. I asked Jesus everyday during my treatments to help me. To give me back my will to live when my will was shallow. I asked Jesus for the strength to be strong and fight. I asked that he give me another chance at my life, so that I can also be an example of his power to help heal.

I wanted so much to have the body he gave me. No disease, no weakness, I wanted to be me again. Run, hike, swim, and play, just like before. I wanted to be like everyone else again not having to think about my illness. Unfortunately, it was only getting worse.

Finally it came time for me to call on mom. Josh and I both agreed that we needed her to come now, spend some time with us before I started getting worse.

It was important for me that she see me as a fighter and not as her very sick child. I wanted her to report the good things back to the family, not that her daughter was very sick and could barely hold her own.

On the day Josh and I were to pick up my mom at the airport, I was feeling sick again. We went to my treatment and the doctors prescribed a stronger pain medication for me to take. I took the medication on the way home from treatment.

As I was anxiously waiting for the time that we were to leave for the airport, I started getting violently ill. I started getting dizzy, vomiting, and breaking out in hives.

I was having an allergic reaction to the medication.

Off to the emergency room we went, yet again! They gave me a couple of shots to calm the reaction down and put me on a heart monitor because the adverse reaction causes a rapid heart rate in some patients.

Josh had to leave me there at the hospital and drive an hour away to the airport to pick up my mom. He didn't want to leave either. It took a nurse to finally push him out the door to go pick up my mom. I felt so alone and scared. I wanted so much to go with him; instead I had to wait in a cold and lonely room feeling scared and sick all by myself.

One of the nurses who realized what was going on came in to talk with me. Her name is Elizabeth. She is a Swedish woman with a warm caring and gentle smile. She sat and talked with me and sang a song in her

Swedish language, that even though I didn't know the words, the song was so sweet, and calming. After I stabilized again I got to go home with mom and Josh.

Mom is staying here for about ten days. Josh and I will show her all around our town and in Florida. She loves the weather here and we have a lot of fun things planned. We want to walk along the beach and collect seashells and looking at the waves crashing against the shore.

For me, the ocean brings a real true sense of Peace, serenity, and fulfillment. I always feel so alive and full of spirit being there. The funniest time we had with mom was when we went to an outside mall over looking the ocean. There was a man with a hotdog stand selling hotdogs. At this time I was unable to eat solid foods. All I could do was take in a DEEP breath and enjoy the hotdogs that way. Josh and mom were laughing so hard at me. I was INHALING the hotdogs, and OH how GOOD it was!!!

Valentine's Day and Josh came home with flowers, a card, and a stuffed animal. I can't help but thank God everyday for bringing such a loving and caring man into my life. Mom is going home today also, I am glad we all got to spend a wonderful time together. Even though I still had treatments this was definitely a visit I would never forget. I only wish my dad had been able to come too.

After seeing mom off on her plane home, Josh realized I wasn't feeling well. We went home and I curled up on the couch with a blanket. I figured I just over exerted myself with my mom's visit. The following morning I awoke very ill again. I couldn't even walk. Josh wrapped me in a blanket and brought me to my treatment. The doctor there took one look at me and sent us immediately to the hospital. I was very dehydrated and was unable to keep anything down. Not even with the help of my feeding tube.

I was admitted to the hospital that afternoon. It took seven hours to go from the emergency department to a room on a floor. I was seen by an infectious disease specialist to help get the blisters and bad infection in my mouth under control. I spent the next several days trying to get better. My treatment was postponed while I had been in the hospital; they felt I needed to regain my strength before they continued.

Josh stayed by my side and read books to me. He helped me in every way he could. At night he slept in a lounge chair right beside my bed incase I needed anything at all. He is definitely my hero, my strength, and my everything.

Many friends and family have been sending Josh and I scriptures and healing prayers to help show their support. I am getting mail from churches, and friends of my parents sharing their experiences and trying to shed some goodness into our thoughts. We are very thankful to everyone who has been praying, caring, laughing, and crying with us. The support is so strong I think everyone we meet can feel the love and strength through us.

The radiation is affecting me more than the doctors could have ever anticipated. I am so sick with vomiting, headaches, mouth sores, and pain in my whole body. I don't know what else to do.

The doctors in the hospital also realize that I need a different type of supplement for my feeding tube. The boost doesn't have enough of the vitamins and minerals I need. By this time I am weighing 73 lbs.

The medications I am on now include: Zylocain, for numbing my mouth, Prednisone, for the infection, Nystatin, also for the infection, Dyflucan, for the infection, Xanax and Zantac, for depression and stomach pain, Acyclovir, a strong antibiotic, and finally Restail, for sleeping. Talk about feeling like a walking medicine cabinet!!! They also changed my supplement to 50cc of Protain XL every hour.

My positive outlook on life and beating this disease is starting to look like that small star way up in the sky that is too far away to touch. I could wish upon that star all I want, but how many times did those dreams come true before?

I knew one thing, although my attitude isn't where it should be, and all I can do is cry, I know one very important and valuable thing: I DON'T WANT TO DIE! The hardest thing for me is trying to figure out what I am fighting against. Is it cancer, myself, my right to want to live? What!? All I can do is cry. I don't want to die; please God let me stay here with my husband, my family, and my friends. Please just for awhile longer.

Again, I start to pray. Pray very hard is what I did. I asked Jesus for the strength I was in dire need for. I need to feel some peace. I know I am not a perfect Angel, but I know deep down inside, that God wouldn't let me down. He will do what he feels is right for me and my family. The horror is not knowing what the outcome will be.

Finally after nine long days I get to go home. What a comfort to know I will be sleeping in my bed with my husband. Oh—don't worry, treatments start back up AGAIN!!! Despite my better judgement.

I did speak with my oncologist on the phone about my concerns and he assured me that when all is said and done it would be over! This was the best news I have heard all week. Now if only I can get my mind to believe this.

The same day of my release from the hospital Josh and I went to pick up my best friend, Lisa. She was flying in from Connecticut to visit Josh and I. It sure feels good knowing that my best friend has never given up on me even though I have moved far away. We had a wonderful visit too. I felt good during her visit.

The visiting nurse comes by the house once every three days to check on feeding tube, to make sure everything is working properly. I know the machine is… I can't vow for my mind and body though. It is difficult to wake up everyday praying I am having a nightmare. It is also hard trying to be so strong when at times I just want to give up.

Towards the end of February I was able to eat some REAL food again. My mouth and throat started to feel a little better and I was trying solid foods again. Being hooked to a feeding tube was really getting to me. I was only able to drink chicken broth by mouth. So I will always remember the days I can eat solid foods.

I had a boiled hot dog, some plain spaghetti, and some boiled cabbage. It wasn't much but let me tell you, not eating FOOD for three weeks and being on a liquid diet was definitely a great joy!

I was drinking so much chicken broth—believe me, I was feeling as if I were starting to grow feathers and rise at the crack of dawn to start clucking and laying eggs.

My family and friends called periodically to check in on us. I never lie to them. Some days are worse than others. All we can do is pray, wait, and be strong. Faith my friend is the only cure. For me, believing in the power of God and the thought that He will do what needs to be done seems to be the biggest thought on my mind.

By this time I have gotten my weight back up. YES, UP! I am now a whole 87 lbs. That is the best weight yet. The most I've weighed since getting sick. Josh and I were so happy. I haven't felt better. Treatments are almost finished.

Now it was time to fight with the insurance company. They would not pay for the new supplement for my feeding tube. The supplement called Protain XL the insurance company felt wasn't necessary when there was over the counter supplements available.

I was so aggravated. I was weighing in at 67 pounds and needed this supplement. Unfortunately the cost would range about $100-$150 a month for Josh and I to pay out of pocket. We couldn't afford this. Everything started to look hopeless once again.

I couldn't believe that something you can only get by prescription to help you stay alive and the insurance company wouldn't pay for this. They might as well start drilling the holes for my coffin, or better yet, pay for a permanent room in the psychiatric ward. I was definitely loosing my mind over this.

Gee! What a *Food for Thought*, huh? Poor Josh, he was so angry not having understood either why they couldn't help us. We had other things to think about. We couldn't think about how I was going to eat too!

We prayed again, for help! A few weeks later we got our prayers answered again. We received a phone call from the clinic over at the military base. The supplement I needed was being bought on my behalf and would be shipped to our home as soon as the pharmacy received it.

We were so overjoyed we held each other and cried. Josh and I will always be grateful to the people who went beyond the call of duty to help us with yet another hurdle. God Bless.

A few days later, after all the additional stress I had endured I am back in the hospital again. Dehydrated, vomiting, and feverish.

Once again I got the chance to become a **HUMAN PINCUSHION**. My IV has been moved to yet another vein. I am so dehydrated my veins keep blowing out after a few hours.

This time they put me on a narcotic to help control the pain. I was put on Demerol. Let me tell you, I saw PINK FUZZY CHICKENS. That stuff was amazing. They would inject the pain medication through my IV and with a few seconds I saw PINK FUZZY CHICKENS, and... Lights Out!

One of the nurses I had on a previous floor saw Josh in the cafeteria downstairs and asked how I was. She came to sit and talk with me after her long and tiring twelve-hour shift. I can't believe how sweet and nice some of these nurses are. It isn't just a job for them; they really love caring for people.

My doctor's assistant came in with one of those turquoise colored scrubs and a BIG white mask that covered his nose and mouth. I can't describe the fear that had just run through me at that moment. All I could think was **NOW WHAT!!!**

What a relief I got when he told me not to worry, he had a sinus infection and because of my POOR IMMUNE SYSTEM, he has to be careful as to not pass the sinus infection on to me. Believe me, I told him... literally, to feel free to stay as far away as humanly possible. WE ALL GOT A GOOD LAUGH AT THAT!!!

Well, I think one of my greatest joys for that day in the hospital was a phone call I received in my hospital room from my Uncle Carmine and Aunt Norma. I miss them so much. I haven't seen my uncle in about five years. We had such a wonderful conversation.

All in all—I was definitely blessed in my life. When I need a pick-me-up, I am sent just the right Angel for the job. No Angel was ever alike. They are all sent with a specific task. And they are all PERFECT.

As for my husband Josh, he is God's gift to me from Heaven above. He has been very strong and supportive to me. He has never let me down. It is an incredible thought to know that I have someone who loves me so much and to be there in sickness and in health. He has definitely fulfilled that vow. The love we share runs deeper than any river and is higher than any mountain.

While being in the hospital this time Josh and I got the opportunity to meet another nurse. His name was Shane. Shane was a piece of work. He would come and sit with Josh and I when he had time and strike up a conversation. He was a very gentle and understanding person.

It was good to know that when I was in pain he would come right away. He never made me feel childish or foolish, no matter how hard I cried or how miserable I felt. He was always there to give a hug. My talks with him opened new outlooks on my battle with cancer. To him and his wonderful family I wish them all the best this world has to offer.

It takes a special talent to do the things that some of these nurses have to do. It isn't easy to cope with watching people who are very ill or those they befriend who even die. My heart goes out to them, and my every thanks to all they do for Josh and I. God Bless.

On the ninth day, the VAMPIRES were back. Sucking out more tubes of blood that I didn't have. Great news though—I am going home tomorrow! I got to eat some semi-solid foods like pudding, and Jell-O, and they stayed down too. I am starting back up with the radiation treatments again tomorrow. **WHOOPI! HERE WE GO AGAIN!**

I can't wait to go home! I am suffering from severe cabin fever. I feel strong again too. With some occasional pain and discomfort, I can say I feel pretty good. I am very thankful for those good days that come after those bad days. At least it gives me something to look forward to.

Finally, day ten of this cabin fever from hell. I feel great. I do have to go to radiation treatment before Josh can take me home though. When we arrived for treatment, the doctor wanted to talk to us.

UT-OH! Now what! Come to find out, the tumor on the base of my tongue was no longer visible. The radiation was working! It was gone!

Oh God! Tears were flowing now. I can't believe it worked. What a blessing this has been. My last day for radiation treatment will be March 24th. Providing there are no more setbacks.

I was so excited to get this news. I could finally start the countdown to finishing treatments. Little did I realize though, the worst was yet to come. (How much worst could it be?)

I was still on more medication than a pharmacy could list on a shelf, but it was helping take the edge off the pain. I was told the physical damage that the radiation was causing may never subside. OH JOY! I already know that the emotional damage of all this will last the rest of my life.

By now I am staring to look like the chipmunks. Don't request a song though, I still can't sing. My whole face was so swollen that I lost the only dimple I had since birth. **RATS!** I really love that dimple. It gave me character. Maybe it was just taking a short vacation, and once the swelling went down it would return. A little wishful thinking never hurt.

I am almost through with my second week of March. The countdown has begun. Unfortunately so has the countdown on my weight. I am now weighing in at 74 pounds and dropping. I can't eat solid foods again and it is back to using the feeding tube.

My face and neck are so swollen that talking has become unbearable. Josh went out and bought me a writing pad and pen to use for communicating. He would talk and relate what I would write when family or friends called the house to check on things. The blisters in my mouth and throat were very bad once again. This time the pain medicine was giving me very little relief.

I was worse than ever, pain, fever, I didn't know what to do. Nothing helped. The strangest thought popped into my head. A young child, somewhere in the world, is going through something similar to me. They have to endure the same kind of pain, if not worse than what I am going through right now. All of a sudden the tears started to fall.

The greatest gift a sick child has is their spirit. They are full of life and inspiration. I thank God everyday for this eye-opener. I am glad that I have become a person who cares about life, and the people who live in it. I am no longer a selfish, non-caring person, who's attitude was her only friend.

There is tragedy in everyone's life. The secret is to overcome it and learn from it. To survive tragedy only makes us stronger in body and mind. I think the saying goes: *What doesn't kill us only makes us stronger*. It really does.

I still have a long road ahead of me. Even after surviving radiation treatment. I still have to have surgery. That shouldn't be so bad though. An incision to cut out that lump. No problem. (Again, little did I realize what was in store for me.)?

Within a few days the fever had gotten to 103 and I was vomiting profusely. It was off to the hospital again. The blisters in my mouth and throat were more infected than ever too. The medication was not working anymore to fight the infection.

My veins were so weak from being dehydrated again that I had several IV's done in just a short time. I was black and blue all over too from the veins collapsing. It was time to be put on another Demerol drip for pain control. (More PINK FUZZY CHICKENS) **Lights Out!**

This time seems to be the hardest on Josh too. I've been sick before but this time is defiantly the worse. He couldn't eat or sleep. He couldn't even bare the thought of leaving the hospital without the fear that I would not be here when he returned. I am so grateful for him. This time was hard. I took 3 steps forward to recovery and 5 steps back in illness.

Again, I was more depressed than ever before. The radiation doctor felt that since I was so close to finishing my treatment and since I was already in the hospital, we would continue treatment. He felt my being in the hospital was the best choice right now.

I was experiencing severe dizzy spells, and vomiting. I couldn't tell who was coming and who was going. I really want to quit! I can't do this! Just make it stop! Please God just make it stop! I tried I really did, but now I can't try anymore. **I can't fight! I am tired!**

When I cried to Josh about giving up, he put me right in my place in a hurry. He told me that he loved me too much to let me die. He couldn't live without his wife by his side. He made it clear to me that I was his everything.

On a funnier note, he told me that because he was in the military, he felt he had rank over me, and that I would need his permission to die… and he wasn't giving it to me! He told me I must fight. We have a long life we have to live together. We have dreams to fulfill and memories to make. He was right!

March 31, 2000. My prayers were finally answered. I was still in the hospital but, I was finishing my last dose of radiation today!!! **Oh God! Thank you! It is finally over!** The tears running down my face were as hot as fire yet as sweet as a spring rain. I did it. I made it to the end.

At the treatment center I got an award from the doctors that they gave to all their *GRADUATING* patients. Everyone was in tears. The doctors, and the nurses. I believe even the ambulance guys that brought Josh and I to the treatment center was crying a little too. This was a touching moment for everyone. A very long time coming, yet a bittersweet goodbye.

On April 3, 2000, after a long two weeks in the hospital, I finally got to go home. I was still sick from the sores, but in time they will heal. The doctors said that the radiation side affects and the precautions I would have to take to help in the healing process could take up to a year to complete. Talk about a very long road! I guess it was for the best that I didn't realize just what was going to happen during treatment. Who knows, I might have just said no. Then again, I wouldn't be here today if I had said no.

I still have a long road ahead. I figure, hey, the worse is over. I would have the strength to keep on fighting. I was gonna be a winner after all. Besides, I make a real bad **LOSER!**

I already made it this far, and how sweet it is to know this is almost over. (So I thought!)

A few days later, I ran into another hurdle on my way to recovery. (I would be crazy to imagine that I wouldn't have anymore hurdles at all). I started vomiting again. It was coming on fast, and furious. I was starting to not be able to hold anything down again. **Not Again! Please!**

I went back for my first follow-up with the radiation treatment center. (FOLLOW-UPS ONLY!). I had another bad infection and was running another fever of 102. I ended up back in the emergency room again. They gave me medication to keep me from becoming dehydrated and medication to control the vomiting. Later that night they sent me home.

The following morning I was given a primary care doctor on the military base that could follow my recovery. It was easier to have a single doctor that knew my history than to see any doctor that wouldn't know what was going on. My doctor took the time to do a complete check-up. I thought she did a wonderful job. She was very competent and thorough. I was glad to see she cared about what was going on.

The doctor ordered a chest x-ray and an abdominal x-ray. She was very determined to see why I was running a high fever. The chest x-ray showed that my lungs were perfectly clear. However, the abdominal x-ray showed some blockage. All the medication was causing a bowel blockage that was causing my vomiting and high fever.

Later that evening after taking the proper medication to relieve the blockage, I felt much better. The fever subsided and I was able to hold some liquids down. Within a couple of days I was feeling pretty good again.

By mid April I was feeling great. (At that time my feeling great was like a normal person having a severe sinus infection—you're not great but you're not that bad either). I still had my good days and bad days. The good were becoming a little more frequent. As far as my eating was concerned I was still using the feeding tube and taking liquid only by mouth.

Back to becoming a chicken again (broth), but now I had a variety. One day chicken broth, one day beef broth. Hey, that was better than nothing. I went back to see my oncologist again to discuss the upcoming surgery. He used the procedure with the tube through the nose and saw no more tumor.

Surgery will be set for May 18, 2000. My mom would be flying in to be support for Josh and me. Now I was starting to see that light at the end of the tunnel. It has been a long time coming, and now I can finally see it. By now I have come to some terms with my Cancer, but never in a million years would I have thought about what I would have to do to fight it. I knew of other people having Cancer, but never imagined the kinds of sacrifices that had to be made.

I am going to be taking part in an event known as <u>RELAY FOR LIFE.</u> This event is a special event that happens in many different states. The event helps the **AMERICAN CANCER SOCIETY** to raise money in the fight against Cancer. I have never been to this event before, yet I have heard a lot about it. This time I will be joining a team.

The day of the event, I ended up in the military medical center. I was showing signs of dehydration, and severe shaking. I was not feeling so good. Everyone at the center knew I wanted to be in the Relay that evening. After a couple hours Josh took me home to rest. That evening we went to the Relay. I was still very sick.

The Relay was very emotional for both Josh and I. They paid tribute to all the cancer victims and survivors. Josh walked with me for my very first SURVIVOR lap. This was the first lap of the Relay. It was designated for all the Survivors. We started out and about mid way through a friend of ours helped Josh with getting me around the lap. I was the last one to cross the finish line, but I DID IT! Josh and I cried, I did the lap, I am a survivor.

I was really sick for most of the evening, and before they even started lighting the luminary bags, I started vomiting. Josh had to take me home. I was so upset. I wanted to stay, but knew I was in no condition to be there any longer.

Lying on the couch at home, I started with severe, uncontrollable shaking. I couldn't sleep. I found that lying down on the cool linoleum floor or sleeping in a warm bath made me feel better. At times Josh had to drive me around in the car for a couple of hours to get the shakes to stop long enough for me to get a few hours sleep.

I had gone back to my oncologist again to explain what was happening. He knew the diagnosis immediately. **WITHDRAWL!** People who are put on narcotics for pain control for a long period of time, and are not weaned off the drugs slowly go into severe withdrawal. The pain and reaction due to the radiation put me in the hospital so many times that I had to keep taking the only medication that could control the pain. **DEMEROL.**

I was on this narcotic for three months before they took me off. **COMPLETELY!** The oncologist said the only hope was to check into a Detox facility. This would be better than what they call an outpatient Detox because I needed to be strictly monitored due to high fevers and poor blood pressure. My oncologist made the arrangement and got me checked in. We needed to straighten out the withdrawl before my surgery.

I was very emotional. With the stress of the cancer, withdrawal, and feeling like I was a drug addict, I couldn't bare it. It was hard to imagine the kind of things the body could do to make you feel so horrible. I just wanted this all to be over!

Josh was only allowed to see me for a couple hours every day. He was even getting nasty at some of the nurses about this. Unfortunately there was nothing we could do. He would call me every chance he got though. Sometimes we talked for awhile, so long as no one else needed to use the phone. Some nurses were very understanding and allowed Josh to stay a little longer during our visits. I felt like a prisoner in that facility.

It had been almost six months of living in pure hell, finished with all the treatments and the Detox. Although I strongly believe that Jesus carried me through some of those bad stages. I was finally free for a short while before surgery. I was able to start eating some semi-solid, yet, very bland foods.

I guess the greatest achievement is to actually want to survive through all that. Wanting to fight. The emotions are definitely the roller coaster ride from hell, but you do learn to adjust, cope, and heal.

Looking back right now I can imagine the torment this put on my husband. The fears, pain, and wonder. Through it all though, our relationship as husband and wife has flourished into a beautiful thing. I don't think we would trade **that** for anything. We have a very strong bond, and I love him so.

CHAPTER 5

May 17, 2000. The day before my surgery. My mom is flying in and I can't wait to see her. After these long and agonizing past couple of months, she will be a sight for sore eyes.

We all went to the oncologist's office to do what is known as a pre-operation work-up. This is where they draw blood, weigh you, take your temperature, and do any additional x-rays needed for surgery. I was told that the incision for my surgery would go from under my chin down my throat about two inches and cut over to the left side of my neck and up behind my left ear. He describes it as a SMILEY face. **WOW!** A lot more dramatic as I would have liked it to be. The procedure is called Lymphatic Dissection.

After we left the oncologist's office I had only one thing left that I could do... I declared the rest of the day as... FUN DAY!

I was tired and weak, but I still had to go out and have fun. We all went to play miniature golf, and fed the alligators. It was a perfect day. The sun was shining and the air was warm, it was such a beautiful day.

Later in the evening, sitting by myself, looking up at the stars, I realized something... I'm really scared. I can't imagine what kind of disfiguration I am going to have after this surgery. Is my husband still going to love me if I look like a freak? I am so terrified. How is the surgery going to affect the rest of my life? I prayed to have some peace about my fears.

May 18, 2000. I didn't get much sleep last night. I have to keep some kind of good composure for my mom and for Josh so they wouldn't worry. It is 6:30 a.m. and we are on our way to the hospital. I can't begin to describe the feelings of anxiety and fear running through my blood at this moment.

The worst part is not knowing how long it would take after the surgery to find out if I have anymore cancer. Not knowing if it has already spread through the lymph nodes and is traveling to other major parts of my body. This is a terrifying thought. Would it be over, or is there another fight I will have to conquer to win? Again, I prayed to God to help me control my deepest, darkest fears.

I sat in the waiting room for my turn to put on, yet, another pair of awful looking booties, and a green cap and gown. As I waited it seemed my life flashed before my eyes. It all happened in such slow motion, yet went by so fast. I can't believe how incomplete life can feel if you don't take the time to stop and view the simple things around you. Life is too short. Enjoy every moment of it. It was time, time for the inevitable surgery. The surgery should last about two hours.

Four hours later, I awoke to find Josh and my mom besides me. I was taken to my own private room. I had a very RUDE AWAKENING! I couldn't breathe. Apparently the swelling was so bad that the bandages around my incision were cutting off my air supply. The nurses had to quickly get the doctors permission to remove the bandages.

A few minutes later, I asked for a mirror. I took a deep breath and held the mirror up. I can honestly say… I was HORRIFIED! They used staples to close the incision, and had to put two drains in to help drain the excess fluid from the lymph node tissue that used to be there. One drain was in the back of my skull and the other was on the side of my neck. Josh tried to point out, as he always does, how beautiful I was.

The pain actually wasn't too bad; they had me on a Demerol drip. Except for the two drains putting excessive pressure onto my head I was doing pretty well. I had lost all the feeling on the entire left side of my face from the cheekbone to the shoulder blade and over to my chin up to my nose. The doctor says it was because the cancer had invaded a sensory nerve and the nerve had been damaged. I still had mobility but no feeling. Some of which may return… in time. The stiffness was so bad I couldn't move my head at all.

Mom and Josh spent the night in lounge chairs by my bed. I can honestly say that I slept like a rock. Then again with all the pain medication and sleeping medication I was on at that time, not to mention the anesthesia that was still running through my lungs. I was a happy camper.

The next morning the doctor came to tell us about the surgery. He said that they strongly believed they got all the cancer out. It would take the pathologist a few weeks to test the tissues and get the report back to the oncologist about where we stood with the cancer. More of the **WAIT… WAIT… WAITING GAME.**

Well, this is where the REAL recovery takes place. I am finished. Now I just have to heal. And now it is time for me to see the *PINK FUZZY CHICKENS* again. (more Demerol) **Lights out!**

After three days the doctor came in and removed one of the drain tubes. Thank goodness it was the one in the back of my head! What a relief to have that drain out. The other drain would have to wait a few more days.

Five days later I was still in the hospital and mom was leaving to go back home. Josh left the hospital just long enough to bring my mom to the airport.

The day before I was to leave the hospital (for the last time, I hope), I had the last of the drain tube taken out. **OUCH!!!** That one really hurt. I still had not gotten any feeling back yet either. My left shoulder muscle and my shoulder blade were very painful though.

A little over a week after the surgery, I got to go home. The staples removed about ten days, and what a difference that made. I had to do some therapy on my range of motion, but it was coming along… slowly and painfully.

I must admit I haven't been myself since the surgery. I have a lot of emotions right now that I can't seem to cope with. I am lost, in pain, and feeling like a FREAK. I know I look like one! With all this swelling and the staples in my neck, it is no wonder I don't scare myself when I look into the mirror. All I feel like doing is going from my bed to the couch. And trying to get comfortable is definitely a chore.

At this time the nerves in my neck and head were trying to rejuvenate and were starting to come alive again. One problem, when they do this they cause severe pain messages to through the head and neck. I am still on the narcotics, but trying to remember just what day it is and where I'm at from one minute to the next is making life more difficult. The doctor said this would be a very long, drawn, and painful transition.

GREAT!!! I can't even begin to explain how many emotions are running through me. Between the anger, the hurt, the confusion, and the worry, I can't seem to get things in a bearable perspective.

It is now the beginning of June and I am having my staples removed. I still have no feeling so it doesn't hurt much when anyone touches my neck. Only my shoulder and head have severe sensitivity, and I am still unable to swallow solid foods due to some scar tissue that has grown over the sight of where the tumor was on my tongue.

Josh has decided to take me away on a well-deserved vacation back to Texas. The doctors gave me the ok, and he wanted us to spend some time together before he had to class back up for school again with the military. (Which I remind you, they put him on a temporary leave to be with me)

Josh and I had a wonderful time. We went swimming and went for walks. I can honestly say that I am now starting to feel better. I can finally start being the wife I wanted to be, instead of the depressed irritable person I had become since this whole treatment started. Life couldn't have been any better at this point. I feel the healing has finally started both physically, mentally, and spiritually.

The only thing left to do was await the results of the surgery. To find out whether or not the cancer had spread beyond the lymph nodes. This was a very scary time, but we knew that we could only pray for the best. I don't know if I could honestly go through anymore treatment at this point. I really don't know.

It was June 12, 2000, when I was outside on the porch with josh talking about how wonderful our relationship is, and how very lucky we are to have each other. The phone rang and I was told it was the oncologist's office calling with the results of the surgery.

My hands were shaking so badly I had a hard time picking up the phone. My mouth felt like I had just chewed up a cotton ball and I couldn't get out a simple word. Finally, after getting my composure back I said hello.

The nurse was on the line and was explaining to me how they don't normally give reports over the phone, however this was important and they knew I was in Texas for awhile visiting family. The nurse advised me in just a few words…

CANCER FREE!!! ALL CLEAR!!! CANCER IS IN REMISSION!!!

I can tell you that the tears fell down my face with total joy. I told Josh and his family and we all just sat there and cried. This was a relief of about 20 pounds off my shoulders. And I know it, meant a lot to Josh too.

You could probably guess that the bells were ringing all over the US that day. We called everyone who had been praying and waiting for the news. It was a day for celebrating and reflecting on our future.

Maria M. Godwin

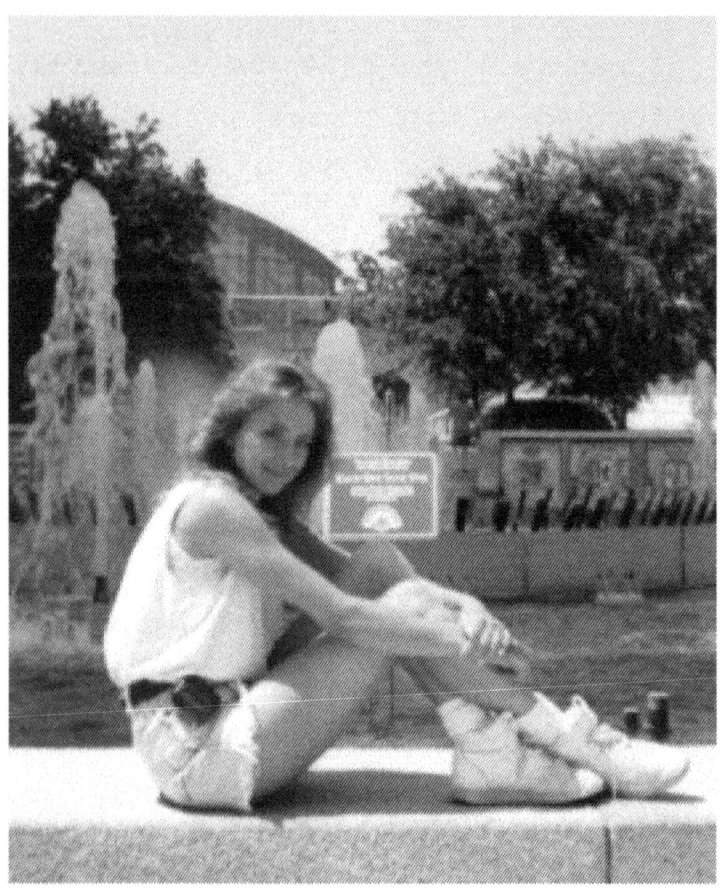

Taking time to visit friends in New Orleans in the summer of 1997.

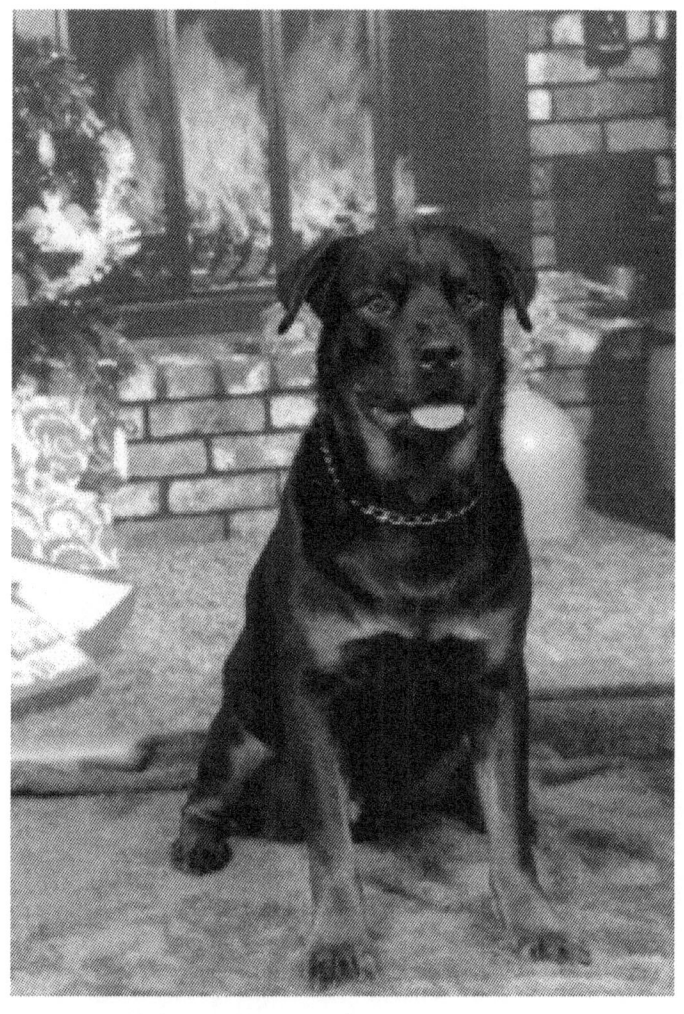

My loyal and faithful friend, Rox in 1997.

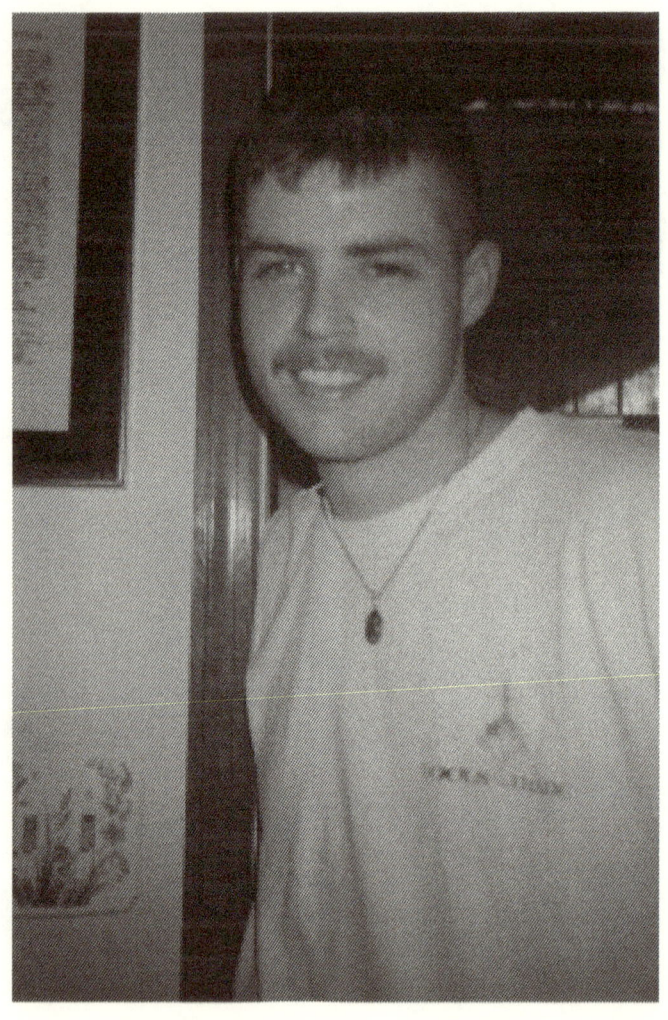

My wonderful and loving husband Joshua.

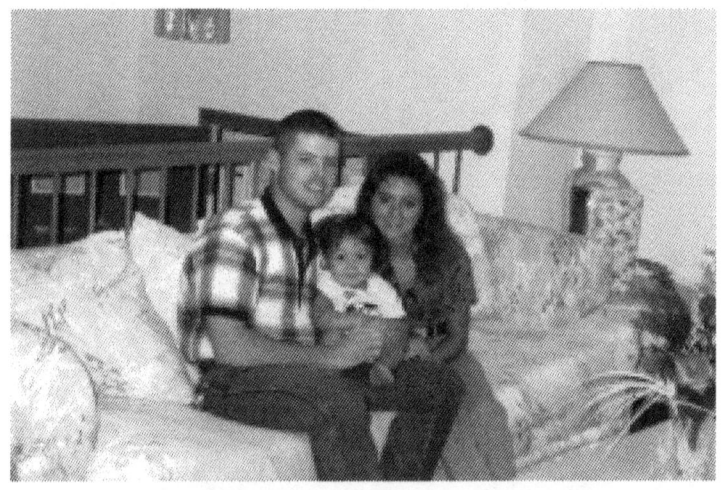

Joshua and I with niece Hannah just before our marriage in August 1999.

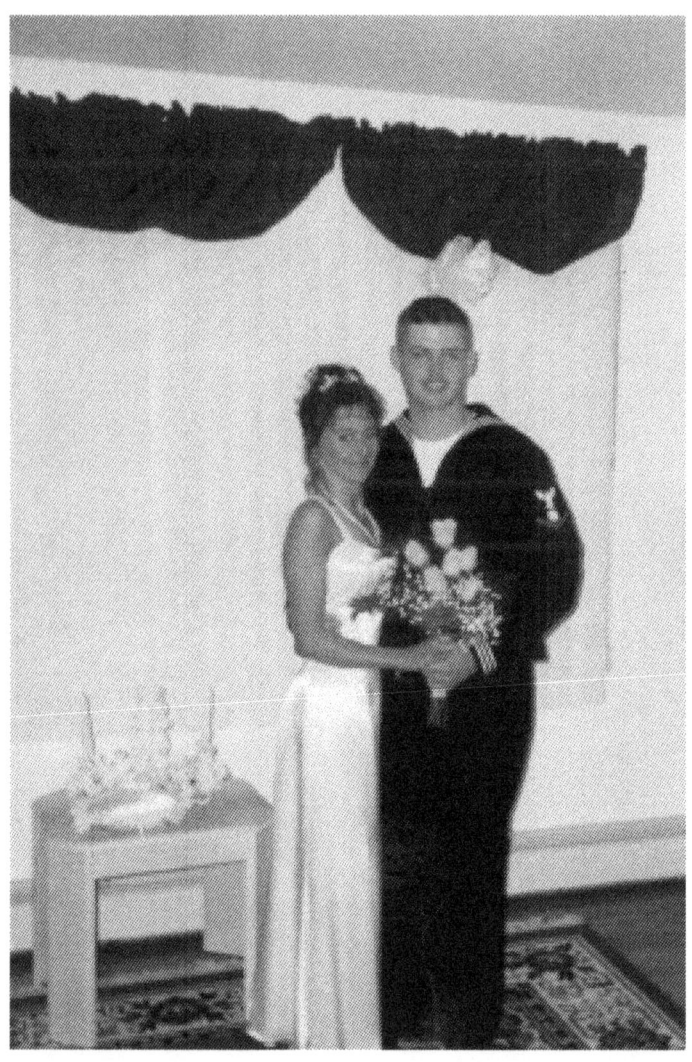

Joshua and I on our Wedding Day.

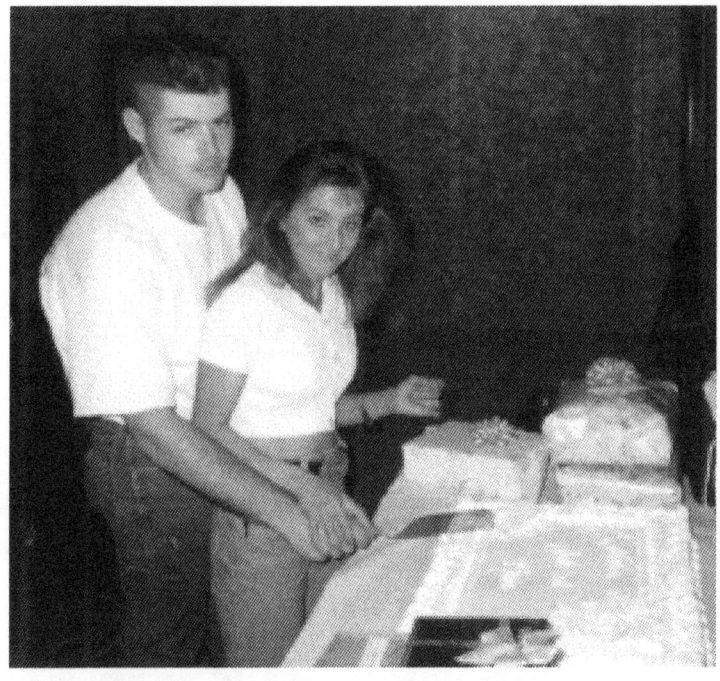

Celebrating our wedding in Texas with family and friends.

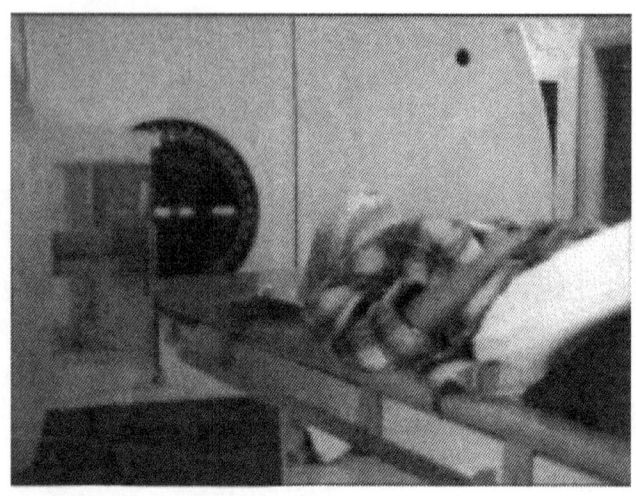

Photos taken just before radiation
treatments started. Mask gets put on
face and then bolted down to table.

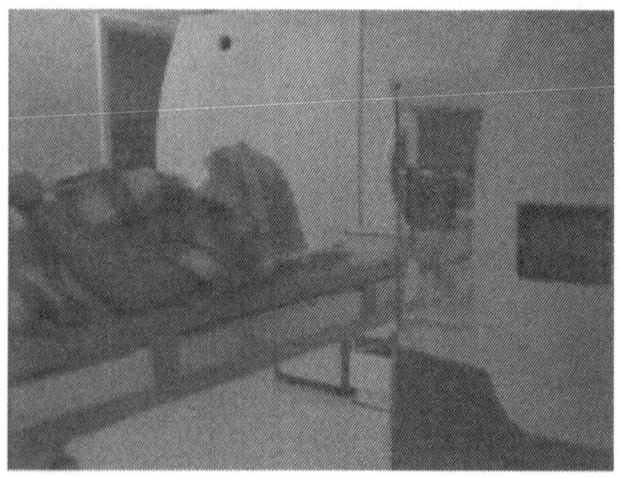

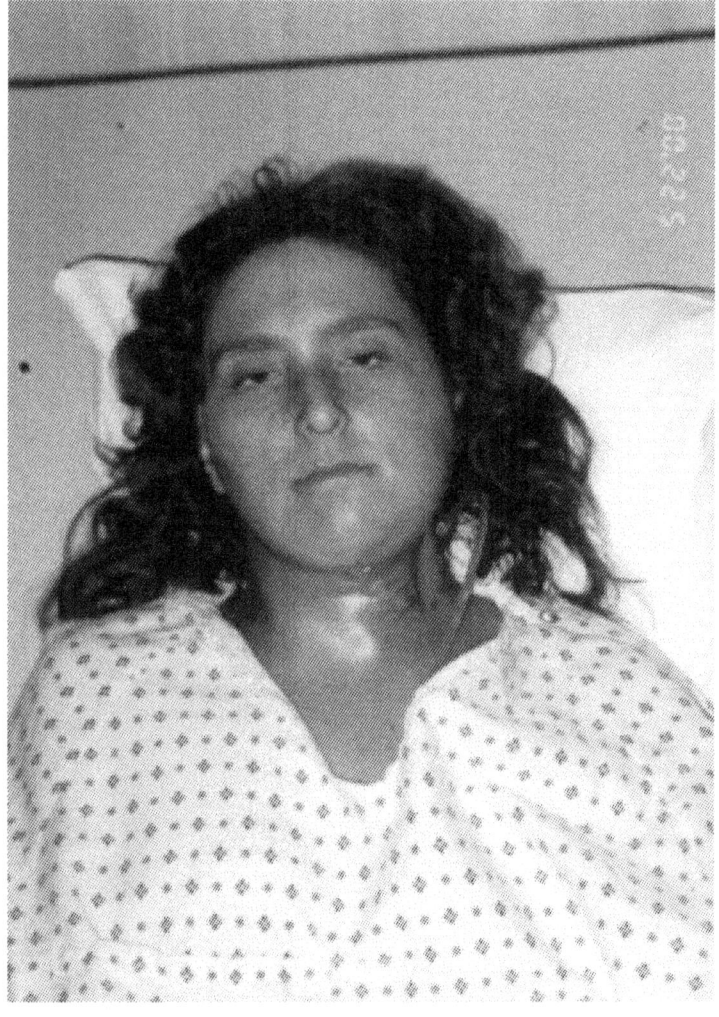

Four days after radical lymphmatic dissection surgery for cancer.

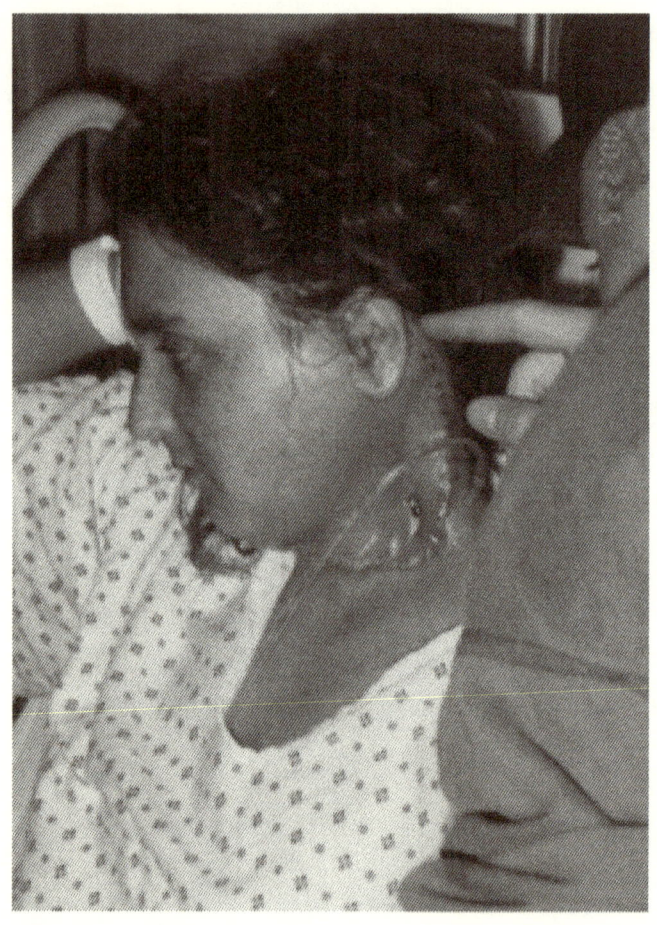

Photo shows swelling of face and drain tube. Also shows where incision and staples were put in place.

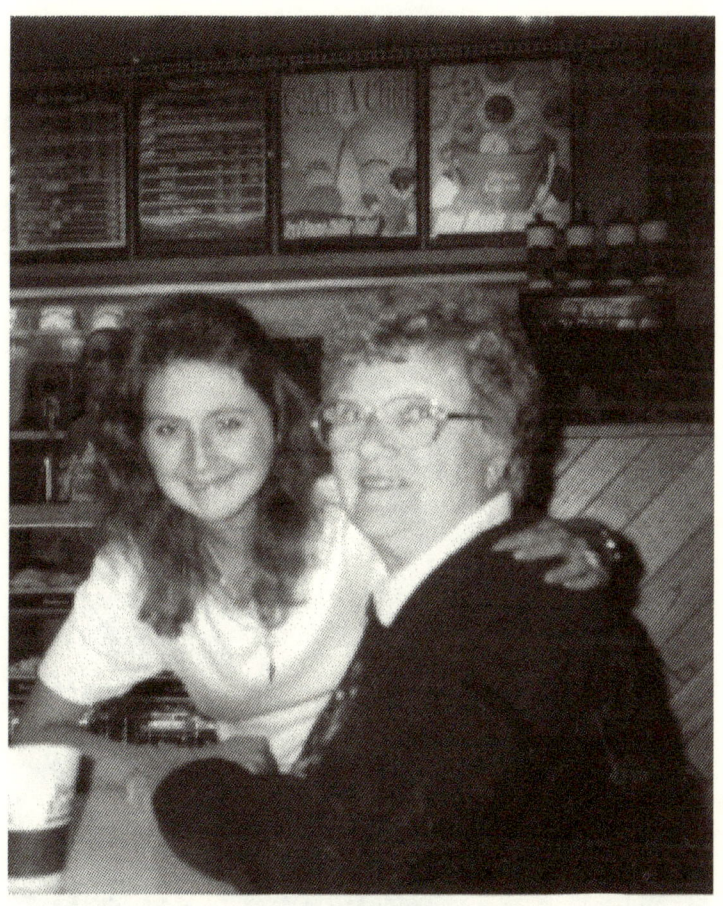

Me with dear friend back home in Connecticut just 3 months after surgery.

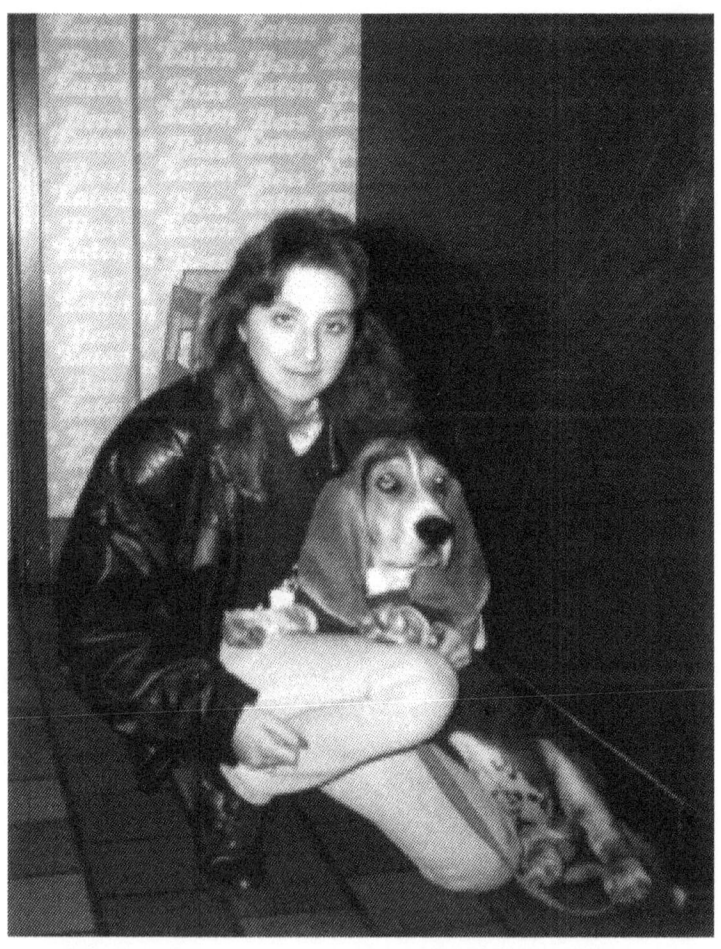

Me and dog, Fred back home in Connecticut 6 months after surgery.

CHAPTER 6

June 20, 2000. Back in Georgia, Josh finally classed back up again. I am healing well from my surgery and starting to feel like my old self again. I still have my feeding tube but the doctors are expecting me to get it removed by October.

I am aware that my chances of another type of cancer to occur are 4%. I have another goal set for me right now, and that is to beat my remission date. May 18, 2002. If I have no recurrences by then my cancer has a 25% chance of never returning. I know this still seems like a lot, but I am alive.

This has been a very challenging year in both my life and Josh's, and I am thankful it is finally over. There are so many people that we need to thank. The prayers and gifts of love and hope were tremendous. A simple thank you still wouldn't seem enough.

All I can say to all our family, friends, and people whom we never even knew, but never the less kept us in their hearts and prayers God Bless. Thank you all for being the strength that Josh and I needed to get us through those difficult times. With you all by our side, we were able to keep the strength and courage; we needed to fight this long and difficult battle.

I don't think I could put into words all the feelings that I am experiencing. I mean for what seemed like an eternity, the cancer, being sick all the time, and the worry if I was going to beat this. To finally hear that I was in remission was almost like hearing that you won something.

I did win something, something more special than any material thing in the world. I won a second chance to make a difference in my life. To live my life to the fullest and to see all the beauty that life has to offer. This is a gift I will never take for granted again.

I now can look at an ocean and smell the salty water. I feel the wind on my face as if it was an Angel lightly brushing my cheek with its wings. I see the mountains in all their majesty. I look at the sky and see the sunshine through the trees while glitters of gold shine on the rippling streams at my feet. So many things we all take for granted. I am now blessed with the opportunity to stop and enjoy life.

Thank you God. Forever and ever, AMEN!

EPILOGUE

2001

Here I am now, 5 months shy of my 2 years of being cancer free. I have to say that looking back into my experiences in my life and how my life is today, all I can say is Thank GOD!

I had the feeding tube removed and am now able to eat fairly well. I was told I will always have trouble eating some foods such as mustard, ketchup, pickles, and acidic foods, and spices. Due to the radiation treatments my saliva has diminished to a point where I need constant water to keep from choking. Eating many things has become a chore, but I get by.

I also have found that the treatments and the surgery destroyed my thyroid so now I am on a medication to help control this. However, that is all the medication I am on now. I have problems from time to time with severe headaches, but that is not too often. As of today, I am weighing in 75 ½ pounds and am feeling great! I know that doesn't sound like a lot, but believe me I feel **GREAT!**

The only thing I will forever feel hurt about is the fact the treatments have caused me to be sterile. Early menopause has set in and no eggs are being produced anymore. The dreams of my husband and me to have our own children have been taken away from us. After serious thought and many tearful nights, we have decided to adopt. We realize that we have so much love to give, and so much of life to share we want to adopt a child.

I have had a few more scares and probably will continue to have them throughout my lifetime. However, I have learned that life is much too short to be worrying about what might happen. I have learned to live for today and make tomorrow a learning experience for the many days to come.

My relationship with my husband has flourished more now than ever before, and we are looking forward to a great LONG life together. As our saying goes… we love each other more today than we did yesterday, and we will love each other more tomorrow than we did today.

Life will never be exactly what we all want it to be, but I can assure you that with the right outlook on life you will always have the beauty in everything you see and do. You only get one chance to make a difference. The little things are what matter most. So take what you have and make it worth your wild.

The world around you may seem dark and stormy at times, but with a little effort we can all add a little sunshine to someone who desperately needs it. So with this, God bless you all, and remember, we never walk alone, the Angels are always with us. Keep an open mind, and as I have said before, believe in the magic of your dreams.

For it is my belief that if we have no dreams and no real life goals, we don't know how to live. So live well, and live for yesterday, today, and tomorrow!

The End!

ABOUT THE AUTHOR

I was born and raised in a small town just outside of New Haven, Connecticut. It was my mom, my dad, my younger sister and I. I grew up in a wonderful house in a quiet neighborhood with a loving family. Times were tough but we managed. We got through the tough times with love and family.

I was always the athletic type. (All 4' 10" of me) I played softball, volleyball, sang in a choir, and was on a gymnastics team for several years.

In high school, I became a bit of a rebel. I was definitely a handful for my parents. Always did the opposite of what I was told. I wanted to do whatever I wanted, no matter what the consequences. I prayed for a good life but never wanted to do anything to get myself there.

I finished high school. (That was a challenge.) I just expected everything to come easy. Finally one day my dreams came true. I got a great job, and stuck to it. I worked hard and got myself an apartment. Then it happened, I met my husband Joshua. Life was finally about to begin. Today, I am thirty-two years old and feel like I have lived a lifetime. My husband Joshua and I have been together for three wonderful years, and live in a house in a small town in Georgia. We have no children so we stock up on plenty of pets. I have four dogs, Buddy, Nitkita, Fred and Cheyeanne, and three cats, Taz, Mittens, Annie. Josh and I are presently doing some remodeling of our home. We are looking into adopting our first child and would love to have a houseful of them too.

Life for me now has changed quite a bit since my bout with cancer, but I can say one thing for sure. Life goes on. And my husband and I are enjoying it together. Life is too short for worries and hustle and bustle.

So enjoy it while you can. My husband and I now live and wonder if I will ever get cancer again, or if I will make it past remission. We try our best not to dwell on it, but maybe dwelling every so often will keep us in touch with reality and the thoughts of what could happen if we should ever forget how to live. We take the time now to look at the sunsets, smell the flowers and go for those long walks on a warm moonlit night. Life has never been so good.